SIMPLE WAYS TO HELP OVERCOME ALCOHOL:

How to easily stop drinking, become safe and sound. (Guided self help)

Peace Micheal

DEDICATION

This book is dedicated to all those who have witnessed
the healing power of this Book and the person currently reading it.

Table of contents

Introduction

Many people have in the past been misled into thinking that moral or character faults cause addiction. Patients with addiction were routinely mistreated. For many years, the norm in addiction therapy was to confine patients to lodging houses, sober homes, or sanitoriums (also known as mental hospitals) until they "dry out," or go through a drug detox, without any kind of medical care.

We now have a better understanding of addiction. Addiction alters the chemistry and operation of the brain, according to researches. Substance abuse hijacks the reward pathways in the brain, triggering intense cravings. When a person stops taking the drug, painful and perhaps dangerous withdrawal symptoms may manifest. The cravings and withdrawal symptoms make it difficult to break the cycle of addiction.

A person undergoing addiction treatment has a number of treatments and levels of care available to them that are intended to help them recover from their alcohol and drug addiction. Addiction therapy is not a one-size-fits-all treatment; rather, it is typically tailored to meet the individual requirements of each patient. You could feel motivated as you prepare to start an alcohol or drug recovery program, but you might also be uncertain of what to expect. However, I can reassure you that beating alcoholism is quite doable with the appropriate program, mentality, effort, discipline, and prayer.

Addiction (disease model)

The American Medical Association and the American Society of Addiction Medicine are two medical organizations that define addiction as a disease.Similar to diabetes, cancer, and heart disease, addiction is brought on by a triad of behavioral, psychological, environmental, and biological factors. Genetic risk factors influence an individual's likelihood of being addicted by around 50%. The brain and body go through changes that lead to addiction with sustained use of nicotine, alcohol, or other drugs.

Consequences of untreated addiction typically include other physical and mental health issues that need medical intervention. If left untreated, addiction increases over time, becoming disabling and even potentially lethal.

To entirely avoid alcohol and refrain from all vices is the goal of this program. Drinking should be cut out early on in the therapeutic process. People may sometimes make mistakes, but successful people are able to get back up and keep moving forward.

The major goals of addiction therapy are to help people deal with cravings, withdrawal symptoms, and maintain their sobriety.

Chapter 1: Evaluating alcohol consumption and issues

Alcohol has been used extensively across many cultures for ages and is a psychoactive drug with addictive qualities. Alcohol abuse has negative social and economic effects as well as a high burden of illness. Alcohol abuse may hurt not just the user, but also everyone around them, including friends, family, coworkers, and total strangers.

Over 200 illnesses, injuries, and other health issues may be directly linked to alcohol use. Drinking alcohol increases the risk of mental and behavioral disorders, including alcoholism, as well as serious noncommunicable illnesses such liver cirrhosis, several malignancies, and cardiovascular diseases.

Accidental and purposeful injuries, such as those brought on by violent acts, road traffic accidents, and suicide, account for a significant amount of the disease burden associated with alcohol intake. Alcohol-related injuries that are fatal often affect younger age groups.

It has been shown that risky drinking is causally related to the occurrence or consequences of infectious illnesses including HIV/AIDS and TB.

Fetal alcohol syndrome (FAS) and difficulties associated with preterm delivery may result from a pregnant woman drinking alcohol.
Unpleasant issue that will continues long after you have sobered up will be in form of:

- Heart issue

You may be aware of the dangers of blood clots, too much body fat, and high cholesterol. Both are more probable when you drink. Heavy drinkers are more likely to have issues with their heart's capacity to pump blood and may be at a higher risk of getting heart disease, according to research.

- Anemia

When your body doesn't make enough powerful red blood cells to transport oxygen throughout your body, this may happen. As a consequence, you can have inflammation, ulcers, and other problems. If you consume too much alcohol, you can skip meals more often, depleting your body of iron.

- Dgestive problems

Alcohol corrodes things. It could cause nausea and heartburn by irritating the stomach lining. Over time, you can have chronic esophageal, stomach, and intestinal inflammation in addition to ulcers. Furthermore, it could make it harder for your intestines to absorb essential nutrients like thiamine and vitamin B12. Alcohol use may produce a buildup of digestive enzymes in the pancreas, which can culminate in a disease called pancreatitis, or an inflamed pancreas. Something may be affecting your capacity to make insulin, which might raise your risk of getting diabetes.

- Sleep

If you drink too much at night, you might lose consciousness. The quality of your sleep might be affected or interfered with when the sedative effect wears off. Too frequent binges might make it hard to go to sleep and stay asleep. Additionally, it might exacerbate sleep apnea and snore, making it challenging to obtain a good night's rest.

- Cancer

High alcohol intake and several cancers are undoubtedly associated. Alcohol may harm the cells in your mouth, throat, voice box, and esophagus. Intestinal, breast, and liver cancer are possible outcomes. Alcohol may facilitate the entry of carcinogens from cigarettes and other sources into your cells.

- Seizures

If you misuse alcohol for a long period, your chance of epilepsy may rise. After excessive drinking, alcohol withdrawal may potentially cause seizures.

- Gout

This kind of arthritis is brought on by the uncomfortable buildup of uric acid in the joints. Red meat, shellfish, and alcohol, particularly beer and liquor, are foods high in purines, which, if ingested in excess, may lead to gout.

- Infections

Your immune system may have a tougher time fighting off viruses and germs if you drink too much. Furthermore, since the liver produces antimicrobial proteins, it may have an impact on your immune system.

Chapter2: Plans for self-management

The road to rehabilitation is unique for each person and takes a lifetime. According to the Substance Abuse and Mental Health Services Administration, recovery is "a process of change during which people improve their health and fitness, live self-directed lives, and attempt to realize their full potentials. Recovery influences many aspects of a person's life since drug misuse typically has a negative effect in many areas of life (e.g., relationships, career, finances, or health).

There are many strategies for healing. For instance, some persons learn that complete abstinence from all drug use is essential in halting the progression of addiction's symptoms. In other cases, a person with a substance use problem may employ harm reduction techniques and adopt healthy thought and behavior patterns to achieve the "health and well-being" linked to recovery without putting too much emphasis on complete abstinence from all drugs.

- Increasing self-drive(motivation)

Motivation plays a crucial role in alcoholism recovery. Regarding their willingness to modify their drinking habits, both alcohol-abusing and alcohol-dependent individuals may be divided into several "stages of transformation." As a result, academics have had to take motivation's function in the management of addiction and recovery from drug usage much more seriously.

However, during the last several years, academics have been more intrigued by the idea of drive and the part that it plays in overcoming alcoholism. Researches have described several phases of change that a person goes through while changing their behavior. These stages include:

pre-contemplation (not yet considering change)
contemplation (considering change but not acting),
preparation (planning to change), action (changing one's behavior), and maintenance (altering one's way of life to maintain new behavior), provide a fresh look at motivation and the behavior-changing process.

Please take note that others with issues like yours have figured out how to quit drinking. You've mastered the art of drinking. You can alter your habits. At this point, it is more vital to find out how to change than it is to worry about how the drinking began. The objective is to completely abstain from all forms of alcohol use. Early in the course of therapy, drinking should cease.

- self-monitoring and recording

Working with factual knowledge is a crucial component of therapy. Writing down information as it occurs is the greatest approach to getting data. It is challenging to remember details afterward. Everyone makes errors while attempting to reconstruct events from the past, whether they occurred a few days ago or yesterday. When you self-monitor, you keep a daily journal of your drinking-related activities. You'll have a better understanding of what's going on if you keep track of your drinking and desires. You and your partner may use monitoring to find trends in your life. You will better understand the behavioral chains that lead to drinking as a result of your monitoring data. Drinkers who self-monitor their drinking are often startled by how much they are consuming and how their drinking tends to follow predictable patterns. You may better understand how often you have the want to drink as well as what triggers these drives by self-monitoring. In general, self-monitoring will assist you in evaluating your development during the program. drawing a self-monitoring card is advised or u can get on from near by medical store. Discipline is crucial in this situation.

Table

Urges			Drinks		
triggers	Scale	Time	Trigger	Kind of drink	Time
Exited at a birthday party	6	8:00pm	Quarrel with jane	Wine 12%	300pm
Watching a tv	5	7:30pm	Passing through a wine bar	Hot wp%	9: am

Example of table for self monitoring

Be careful to include the date on the card while filling it out. For each day of the week, a card should be filled out. Analyze the data from your cards to find any trends that appear over the week.
Write down the time the impulse happened and how strong it was in the area labeled "Urges." Enter a number between one and ten for intensity to indicate the degree of the desire. Number 1 would indicate a very mild yearning. Number 10 indicates that the need was the greatest you had ever experienced. Give it a number in the center if the desire was in the middle. Note what made you feel the desire.
Drinks: List the drinks you had, how much of them you drank, and their alcohol content in the "Drinks" area. Enter the time you began drinking in the "Time" field.
Continue this sequence week after week, you will then discover a particular trend.
This trend has to be altered at all cost. Develop schedules to run through such period.

- Triggers

Relapsing on alcohol is a risky practice since it may rekindle addiction and lead to overdose and alcohol poisoning.
Strong cravings and drives for alcohol may be brought on by certain individuals, places, objects, and emotions, which may result in relapse.
You may reduce your chance of relapsing and maintain your sobriety by knowing your triggers, comprehending how they relate to cravings, and taking appropriate action.

Addiction is often characterized by very strong cravings for alcohol and other substances. Even years after your last drink, you could start to feel the want to drink again. Though many of these cravings will be brought on by stimuli you encounter daily, others may be irrational.
Learn more about the most typical reasons for alcohol relapse in the next paragraphs, as well as how to prevent relapse by avoiding triggers.

What are alcohol usage triggers, and how do they develop
Anything that conjures up thoughts of drinking or a desire to partake in an alcoholic beverage is a trigger. Triggers might be important and symbolic or they can be something entirely unrelated to your previous drinking that serves as a trigger.

Triggers develop as a result of the brain's training from drug use to pay particular attention to anything related to alcohol. By producing a substance called dopamine, it does this. Alcohol has such a strong and satisfying effect that the brain is always looking for excuses to have another drink. Even if you are in recovery and know that drinking would have bad effects, this still happens.

Relapse may result from cravings, which are triggered by triggers. Knowing your triggers can help you prolong your recuperation. What are the most typical reasons why individuals start drinking again?

Alcohol consumption triggers are often divided into several categories. You may reflect on your problems and create a comprehensive database by doing this, The people, places, and things that you identify with your previous drinking are the most frequent alcohol use triggers. A strong urge to drink might also be sparked by certain emotions and moods.

People: Are they capable of causing a relapse?

The individuals you drank with will probably be the biggest relapse triggers. If you often consume alcohol with friends or family, you could have cravings whenever you see them. People who could make you want to drink include:

-Your siblings, parents, and grandparents -Your little ones
-Your college buddies
-Your superiors and coworkers
-Individuals from the bar you know
-Random drunk individuals
-Those that elicit a powerful emotional response

Some individuals could be aware of their relationship with alcohol. Others, though, can be utterly blind to this. Additionally, not everyone will always act as a trigger. To experience the trigger, many circumstances will need to come into play.

Where may I be more likely to drink?

The locations where you drank the most often are the ones that are most likely to cause an alcoholic appetite. These locations will probably be triggers for you if you usually drank when you went to your friends' residences or a certain restaurant. Some of the most frequent locations that cause alcohol cravings include bars and liquor shops. The mere act of passing by these locations might make you hungry.

Places might be restricted to a certain area of a home or structure. Others could be tempted to drink by a street or a whole city. Triggers are adaptable in terms of geography.

What other things may I desire a drink for?
If your brain has made a connection, almost anything may make you desire to drink. An impulse to drink may be brought on, among other things, by:

-Observing a bottle of booze
-A certain day of the week or hour
-A sweltering summer day or a chilly winter night
-A significant birthday or event
-Receiving money or payment
-Arguments and disagreements
-To observe a sports event
-Substances such as cigarettes, cocaine, or cannabis (marijuana)
There may not always be a direct correlation between the object and your alcohol consumption. The need may be triggered by anything, even if it makes no sense.

How does my mental state or amount of stress affect whether I relapse into drinking?
Your mood may make you want to consume alcohol. The impulse to use alcohol as a kind of self-medication may be triggered by unpleasant feelings and times of extreme stress. Alcohol produces pleasure sensations that lessen the force of these unpleasant feelings.

If you encounter any of the following:

-Angry or Sad
-Angered or displeased
-Anxious
-Bored

-Lonely

It turns out that relapse is also associated with happy emotional states. The need to drink may be sparked by emotions like happiness, excitement, or the need to celebrate.

Alcohol may at times seem to be the sole option for controlling strong or fluctuating emotions. However, drinking prevents you from learning effective coping mechanisms.

What can I do about the causes of relapse

It is crucial to recognize, catalog, and comprehend your alcohol use triggers, but this is just the first step. You must now decide how to lessen the frequency and potency of these triggers. There are just two distinct ways for the majority of individuals to handle triggers:

1) You can either completely dodge the triggers.

2) Alternately, you might provide them with a strong relapse prevention strategy.

How can you prevent triggers and stay sober?

The simplest method to deal with triggers is sometimes to avoid dangerous situations, people, objects, and emotions. You may find that your desire for alcohol is significantly reduced if you can avoid a certain person, location, or circumstance.

The problem here is that certain triggers can't be prevented. A certain number of people, places, and objects must be encountered. Some triggers, such as occasions like holidays, anniversaries, or places, could be impossible to avoid. Additionally, you cannot control certain feelings, such as grief or rage. These emotions sometimes come over everyone.

Examine all of your triggers and divide them into "avoidable" and "unavoidable" columns to determine what you can avoid. Avoid as much as you can and direct your attention to others.

How can you prepare your response to drinking triggers?

One of the most important aspects of alcohol rehabilitation is avoiding relapse. Although there are various methods to maintain sobriety, not all strategies will be effective for everyone. Try out a variety of strategies and find which ones work best for you.

The following are some of the greatest methods to react to triggers:

-Making a call to a sponsor, a loved one, or a mental health professional
-Going to a self-help gathering
-Developing relaxation techniques
-Concentrating on the drawbacks of drug usage, such as the possibility of losing my work. I may get drunk and crash my car. I might endanger my marriage even more. I could put my kids at risk. I may sour a relationship. I might endanger my health even more. I risk losing my family's and friends' respect. I risk losing my respect. I may not take care of my domestic duties. I could exacerbate my drug addiction issue. Instead, think to yourself, "I'll be one step closer to total sobriety." I'll be able to speak with my husband intelligently. I won't have a headache when I awaken. I'll be able to delight my employer by arriving at work on time. I'll get to enjoy some quality time with my family. I'll be in a position to lead by example for my children. I will be able to go securely by car. Savings will be possible for me. I'll be able to take care of my domestic duties. I'll be able to consume satisfying, healthy meals.
-Thinking about the effects of acting on your triggers and "playing the tape"
-Exercising
-listening to music or seeing a movie
Eating a nutritious snack
-The nice thing about these alternatives is that you can use many ones at once. You are not required to choose only one. Relapse prevention strategies are very individualized, so consider and develop your strategy before your subsequent cravings.

Chapter 3: Discipline and prayer

Reward, Inspiration, Discipline and Prayer
Alcoholics and drug addicts have a difficult time adhering to a treatment plan. Motivation fluctuates. Discipline is a distinct concept. It's a deliberate, persistent effort that has been made over time. It requires repetition and the development of positive habits. It takes discipline to stay sober.

But it's crucial to avoid being constrained by regulations. The ultimate goal of discipline in recovery is to get the prize. Freedom is the reward. Keep your sights set on the goal even when things become challenging.

I just can't do it sometimes. I'm having trouble starting the piece I need to be writing. I'm easily sidetracked. Instead, it's a day when I should definitely go for a run. But as I gaze out the window, I decide not to bother. I know what I should be doing, but I simply can't get out of bed. I feel lethargic. There are several defenses. I no longer have the drive. Alcoholics and those with other addiction illnesses may connect to this readily. I was inspired to cut down and become more mindful of my intake after I began to realize that I had lost control of my drinking and it was harming me. I would keep track of how many alcohol units I drank each day for a week. But the euphoria quickly subsided. I have sometimes been able to completely refrain from drinking for days or even weeks, but my old drinking habits always crept back and only became worse. It is very apparent why the military needs strict discipline, but the same is equally true for addicts. Alcoholics often attend treatment with the best of intentions when they are at their lowest point. They are undoubtedly anxious, but they are also driven to recover. Unfortunately, with time, motivation tends to wane and relapse risk increases for the alcoholic.

Discipline may be used to develop positive habits that can take the place of "substance use disorder". Habit is the repetition and memory-based way we think and behave in the environment. We could have a tendency to act morally and in our own best interests. Presumably, we do not consciously decide to engage in detrimental behaviors over and over again. However, our logic is faulty. We often struggle to accurately separate good from negative. When we allow our passions to rule us, we make bad decisions, and our habits show this.

Repetition, an 1843 essay by the Danish philosopher Soren Kierkegaard, addressed the issue of habit. He made the case that repetition throughout time contributes to our "becoming". Through consistent practice, we discover who we are and develop into the people we are. In other words, a habit is a component of who we are. Through our routine behaviors, we let other people in on who we are, at least in part. Developing or modifying our identity as a person entails altering our routine behavior. The controlled practice of habit, either individually or collectively, may sometimes be referred to as "ritual." It is not thoughtless. We may notice the function of ritual when we examine organized religion or spiritual practices. What you do, why you do it, and who you do it with all have meaning, serve as a reminder, and they are communal.

What kind of controlled behaviors are we considering

Here are a few ideas. Pick your favorite non-alcoholic beverage for the dinner party or the beach. Hold on to it. Make your response to being given booze in advance. Prepare your response in case someone inquires as to your reasons for abstaining from alcohol. If you find it useful, you can decide to make a weekly commitment to attend fellowship sessions on a certain day. Make it a routine. Maintain discipline in this.

There are a few more things to consider in this situation. First of all, you cannot improve on your own. Maintaining motivation and discipline on your own is challenging. If you do it with others, it will be simpler. As a result, you may rely on people when you are feeling weak. Others may watch out for you and apply some kind of outward punishment.

Second, make things simple. Avoid being too ambitious. Set some straightforward goals, such as "one day at a time." Don't make it so difficult that you end up beating yourself up for not sticking to it.

Discipline is serving a greater goal, which is another crucial point to keep in mind in this situation. We don't want to live lives that are governed by laws, replacing one type of captivity with another. We have reason to be hopeful in the face of our present suffering because of the promise of recompense. I find it fascinating that some mentees have inquired as to how they may substitute the alleged "prize" of alcohol or illicit substances.

In the end, we might consider the reward to be the prize. Liberation is the goal of addiction therapy. In a broader sense, liberation from all types of captivity is the reward for spiritual well-being. Freedom from being held captive by substances like alcohol or narcotics, material goods, worries about what other people think of us, and uncontrollable fears.

We're competing in a race. Disciplined habits are necessary to boost motivation. We must also keep going till the goal is reached. Focus on the goal at all times!

- Prayers(most important)

The most important but seldom spoken aspect of many programs is the attitude, which has a lasting and direct impact on our mental health.

When faced with a triggering scenario, long-term Alcoholics Anonymous (AA) members find that prayer reduces their want to drink. According to recent research that examined the brain physiology of long-term program participants who were in recovery from alcoholism, this is the case. Following the viewing of drinking-related pictures, those who said the AA prayers reported fewer alcohol cravings and showed higher activity in the parts of the brain that regulate attention and emotion.

A prayer by American theologian Reinhold Niebuhr known as the "serenity prayer" has been adopted by several twelve-step programs, including AA, which uses the following version: God, give me the peace to accept what I cannot alter, the courage to do so, and the discernment to recognize the difference.

Researchers from the NYU Langone Medical Center undertook what is believed to be the first study to look at brain physiology among AA members. 20 long-standing AA members were recruited by the researchers to take part in the study.

These volunteers, who had not had any alcohol cravings in the week leading up to the test, were then put in an MRI scanner and given images of alcoholic beverages or drinking individuals.

The images were presented to each individual twice.

Following the watching in the first round, the participants were required to read objective content from a newspaper.

In the second, they said an AA prayer that encourages alcohol abstinence. All of the study participants claimed to have experienced some level of hunger after seeing the photographs. But after saying an AA prayer, the urge subsided.
Marc Galanter, MD, professor of psychiatry and director of the Division of Alcoholism and Drug Abuse at NYU Langone, is the senior author of the study and its senior author. "Our findings suggest that the experience of AA over the years had left these members with an innate ability to use the AA experience - prayer in this case - to minimize the effect of alcohol triggers in producing craving," he says. "Long-term AA members had lower cravings than patients who have abstained from alcohol for some time, but they are more prone to relapse."
Thirty volunteers who said they had no desire for alcohol the week before the test was chosen by the researchers. They were positioned in an MRI machine and showed images of alcoholic beverages or drinking individuals.
Following the viewing of the photos, every participant stated having some level of desire. Reports of cravings, however, reportedly subsided after saying an AA prayer. The team was also able to identify physical brain reactions using information from the MRI images. We wanted to find out what happens in the brain when long-term AA members are exposed to alcohol-craving cues, like walking by a bar or going through a traumatic experience, Galanter adds.
They argue that this speaks to the many ways in which individuals interpret events depending on their point of view.

According to Galanter, the research "indicates that there seems to be an emotional reaction to alcohol cues, but that it is experienced and understood differently when someone has the protection of the AA experience." For ten years, Galanter has researched the function of spirituality in long-term AA members. He has discovered that this group goes through a "spiritual awakening" that ushers in a change in drinking habits.The length of time that has transpired since this changeover is related to desire reductions.
According to Galanter, "Our latest results open up a new avenue of investigation into physiologic alterations that may follow spiritual awakening and perspective adjustments in AA members and others."

Chapter 4: Management of Mood

- Anxiety

Anxiety is a common feeling. It's how your brain responds to stress and warns you of impending danger.Everybody has occasional anxiety. When confronted with a challenge at work, before a test, or before making a crucial choice, for instance, you could worry.

Periodic anxiousness is okay. Anxiety disorders, however, are distinct. They are a set of mental conditions that produce unrelenting, intense worry and terror. You may avoid activities such as work, school, family gatherings, and other social events because of your extreme anxiety since they might exacerbate your symptoms.

Danger signs for anxiety disorders

-A history of mental illness: Your chance of developing an anxiety disorder is increased if you already have a mental health condition like depression.

-Sexual abuse of children: Childhood sexual, emotional, or physical abuse or neglect has been related to anxiety problems in adults.

-Trauma: A stressful experience raises the likelihood of developing posttraumatic stress disorder (PTSD), which may result in panic episodes.

-Adverse incidents in life: Your chance of developing an anxiety disorder is increased by stressful or unfavorable life circumstances, such as losing a parent when you were a young kid.

-Severe ailment or ongoing medical issue: You may experience overwhelming stress and anxiety if you are constantly concerned about your health, the health of a loved one, or the needs of a sick person.

Addiction to drugs: Alcohol and illicit drug usage increases your risk of developing an anxiety condition. Additionally, some individuals utilize these drugs to mask or lessen their anxiety symptoms.

-Being reserved as a kid: Social anxiety in teenagers and adults is associated with early shyness and retreat from strange people and environments.

-Self-esteem issues: Social anxiety disorder may be brought on by negative self-perceptions.

-Genetics would be an additional influence: Disorders of anxiety may run in families.

-Mind chemistry: According to several studies, dysfunctional brain circuits that regulate emotions and fear may be responsible for anxiety disorders.
A stressful environment: This is a reference to tense situations you have seen or experienced.
-Childhood abuse and neglect, the loss of a loved one, being assaulted or seeing violence, and these types of life experiences are often associated to anxiety disorders.
Drug abuse or withdrawal: Some anxiety symptoms may be concealed or reduced with specific medications. Alcohol and drug abuse can go hand in hand with anxiety disorders.
-Ailment conditions: Some heart, lung, and thyroid diseases may exacerbate or induce symptoms that are similar to those of anxiety disorders.

How to rationalize anxiety problems
Keeping a log

Date	Time	Situation	Thought	Anxiety level
9-04-22	2:30am	Woke up on bed in the nigh	I have got exams 2moro and I haven't covered all syllable	8

An example of how to self record an anxious mind. Include more pattern related to you inorder to observe your body chemistry

Controlling an anxiety condition
-Understand your disease: The more information you have, the better equipped you'll be to deal with symptoms and obstacles along the path. Ask your wife, friend or doctore any questions you may have without hesitation. Keep in mind that you play a vital role on your healthcare team.
-Adhere to your treatment schedule: Stopping your medication abruptly might have unpleasant side effects and can make you feel anxious.
-Reduce your intake of caffeinated foods and beverages such coffee, tea, cola, energy drinks, and chocolate. The mood-altering stimulant caffeine may exacerbate the signs and symptoms of anxiety disorders.
-Don't drink or use illegal substances recreationally. Abuse of drugs raises your chance of developing anxiety problems.

Eat healthily and move more.

-Exercises that are vigorously aerobic, like running and bicycling, help the brain produce hormones that reduce stress and elevate mood.

-Improve your sleep: Anxiety disorders and sleep issues often coexist. Prioritize getting enough rest.

-Establish a peaceful nighttime routine. If you are still having difficulties sleeping, see your doctor.

-Learn to unwind: Your treatment approach for anxiety disorders must include stress management.

-After a stressful day, practices like meditation or mindfulness may help you relax and may even improve the efficacy of your therapy.

-Publish a journal: Before the day is through, try to relax by writing down your thoughts so that you won't spend the whole night tossing and turning with worry.

-Control your negative thinking: Instead of worrying thoughts, it might be beneficial to think happy ones. However, if you have some kinds of worry, this might be difficult. You may learn how to reframe your thinking via cognitive behavioral therapy.

-Get a group of pals together: Social interactions, whether in person, over the phone, or online, support individuals in thriving and maintaining their health. Social anxiety is less common in those who have a tight circle of friends who encourage them and engage in conversation.

-Seek assistance: Speaking with others who are going through the same things may be motivating and useful for some individuals.

-Self-help or support groups provide you the opportunity to discuss your issues and accomplishments with others who understand.

Before using any over-the-counter medications or herbal cures, consult your doctor or pharmacist. Many include substances that might exacerbate the feelings of anxiety.

- Depression

What Is Depression

It takes more than simply feeling sad or having a terrible day to be depressed. You may be depressed if a depressive state persists for a long period and interferes with daily activities. Depression symptoms include:

-Feeling depressed or worried often or always
-Not wanting to engage in previously enjoyable activities
-Feeling easily aggravated, angry, or restless
-Having issues sleeping or staying asleep
sleeping excessively or waking up too early
-Eating more or less than usual, or not being hungry
-Aches, pains, headaches, or gastrointestinal issues that don't go better with therapy
-Unable to focus, recall specifics, or decide what to do
-Despite getting enough sleep, you still feel exhausted
feeling useless, guilty, or powerless

Considering harming or killing oneself

The following information cannot replace consulting a mental health professional and is not meant to be a medical diagnosis of serious depression. Talk to your doctor or a mental health professional right away if you believe you are depressed. This is particularly crucial if your symptoms are worsening or interfering with your everyday activities.

Why Do People Get Depressed

Depression's precise origin is uncertain. A confluence of genetic, biochemical, environmental, and psychological elements may be to blame. Although every individual is unique, the following things may make someone more likely to experience depression:

-Having family members that have experienced depression
-Experiencing painful or stressful situations, such as being subjected to physical or sexual abuse, losing a loved one, or facing financial difficulties
-Undergoing a significant shift in one's life, even if it was planned
-To have a medical condition like cancer, a stroke, or persistent discomfort
Taking certain medicines, If you are uncertain as to whether your prescription drugs are contributing to your depression, see your doctor.

Who Develops Depression

On average, 1 in 6 persons will experience depression at some point in their lives.

Every year, nearly 16 million adult Americans suffer from depression. Anybody may experience depression, and it can strike at any age or in any sort of person.
In addition to having depression, many individuals also have other mental health issues. Depressive illnesses and anxiety disorders often coexist. Anxiety disorders cause severe and uncontrolled sensations of anxiety, dread, concern, and/or panic in its sufferers. These emotions may last for a long period and might obstruct regular tasks.

What Medicines Are Used to Treat Depression

There are several effective therapies for depression. Depression treatment may help lessen symptoms and cut down on how long it lasts. Getting treatment may include going to counseling or taking medication. The optimal course of therapy for you may be decided with the assistance of your doctor or a certified mental health expert.

Therapy. Psychotherapy, which is also known as therapy or counseling, helps a lot of individuals. The majority of therapy sessions are brief and concentrate on the problems, emotions, and ideas that are currently going on in your life. Understanding your history might be helpful in certain situations, but figuring out how to deal with what is going on in your life right now can help you cope and be ready for problems in the future. In therapy, you'll work with your therapist to develop coping mechanisms, alter problematic habits, and come up with solutions. Talking freely and honestly about your thoughts and worries is not anything to be ashamed of or bashful about. Gaining improvement requires doing this. Among the typical objectives of treatment are:
-Becoming more healthy
giving up smoking and abstaining from drugs and alcohol
-Overcoming phobias or other concerns
Managing stress
Understanding tragic historical occurrences
recognizing the factors that make your sadness worse
-Improving communication with family and friends
-Knowing the source of your annoyance and making a strategy to deal with it
-Medication: Antidepressant medicines are often administered to persons with depression to help them feel better and develop better coping mechanisms. Ask

your doctor whether they are appropriate for you. Ask your doctor for specific instructions on how to take the antidepressant if they prescribe it to you. Tell your doctor if you are already receiving nicotine replacement therapy or another drug to help you stop smoking. You and your doctor have a selection of antidepressant drugs to choose from. Be patient; it may take a few attempts to discover the ideal drug and dosage for you. Moreover, remember the following crucial details:
-It's crucial to take these prescriptions as prescribed, so pay attention to the dosage guidelines. Some patients feel better a few days after taking the drug, but the full effects may not be felt for up to four weeks. The majority of individuals find antidepressants to be effective and safe, but it is still vital to discuss any adverse effects with your doctor. The majority of the time, side effects are not bothersome and disappear as your body becomes used to the drug.
-Avoid stopping an antidepressant without first seeing your physician. Sudden medication withdrawal might exacerbate depression or trigger symptoms. To safely modify your dosage, see your doctor.
Some antidepressants include dangers when used while pregnant. If you think you may be pregnant or if you want to become pregnant, discuss it with your doctor.
All of your issues cannot be resolved with antidepressants. Calling your doctor immediately away is crucial if you find that your mood is deteriorating or if you have suicidal thoughts.

Finding Support During a Crisis with Depression and Suicide

When sad, some individuals consider harming themselves or killing themselves (taking their own life). Please seek urgent assistance by getting in touch with your therapist if you or someone you know is considering harming themselves or taking their own life.

Qestion and self management Plans

What circumstances are likely to make you feel down
• Waking up at 4 or 5 a.m.
• Difficulty focusing • Change in appetite • Moving slowly
• Feeling worthless or having poor self-esteem
• Fatigue or lack of energy
• Feelings of despondency

What kinds of ideas are likely to make you feel down?
When you're sad, how do you feel?
What relieves your depression the best?
Keep in mind that although drinking may provide a little reprieve from melancholy and depression, over time it only serves to exacerbate the condition and to develop new issues that, in turn, may contribute to depression. You will discover a way out of the vicious cycle with the assistance of your therapist.

- Anger control

According to Charles Spielberger, Ph.D., a psychologist who specializes in the study of anger, anger is "an emotional state that ranges in intensity from moderate annoyance to severe wrath and violence." Similar to other emotions, anger is accompanied by physiological and biological changes. For example, when you feel furious, your blood pressure, heart rate, and levels of the chemicals adrenaline and noradrenaline all increase.

Events both internal and external might trigger anger. A traffic delay, a flight cancellation, or a particular person or incident might be the source of your rage, or it could be brought on by fretting or obsessing over personal issues. Anger sentiments may also be sparked by memories of upsetting or painful experiences.

Responding violently is the automatic, natural manner that anger is expressed. Anger generates strong, often violent sentiments and actions that enable us to fight and protect ourselves when we are attacked. Anger is a normal, adaptive reaction to danger. Therefore, some level of rage is essential for our existence.

On the other hand, laws, societal conventions, and common sense impose boundaries on how far our rage may lead us. As a result, we can't physically strike out at every person or thing that frustrates or annoys us.

People cope with their anger sentiments in several conscious and unconscious ways. The three major strategies are calm, inhibit, and express. The best method to deal with anger is to express it in a confident, non-aggressive manner. To do this, you must learn how to express your demands and how to meet them without harming other people. Respecting yourself and others requires being forceful without being aggressive or demanding.

Anger may be contained, then transformed, or directed. This occurs when you suppress your rage, put it out of your mind, and concentrate on the good. Your anger is to be contained or suppressed to channel it into more useful activity. If your anger isn't permitted to find an outlet outside of yourself, it might move inside and toward you. Anger that is directed inside might result in sadness or high blood pressure.

Anger that goes unspoken might lead to other issues. It may result in pathological outbursts of rage, such as passive-aggressive conduct (attacking others covertly without explaining why rather than outright) or a persistently angry and cynical mentality. People who continuously belittle others, criticize everything and make cynical remarks lack the ability to vent their anger in healthy ways. They are unlikely to have many fulfilling relationships, which is not unexpected.
You can now settle down inside. This entails managing both your external conduct and internal reactions, slowing down your pulse rate, calming yourself down, and allowing the emotions to pass.
"When none of these three strategies succeed, that's when someone or something is likely to be wounded," observes Dr. Spielberger.

Anger management aims to lessen the physiological stimulation that anger creates as well as your emotional sentiments. You cannot alter, ignore, or get rid of the things or people who irritate you, but you can learn to regulate your emotions.

Some quick strategies to help you understand and control your angry behavior

To determine the circumstances that make you angry, use the worksheet on anger triggers included in this chapter. Then, choose a trigger from the worksheet on anger triggers, and complete the worksheet on the anger behavior chain for that trigger.
Thoughts/Feelings Column: Write down your thoughts when you last encountered this trigger and think back to that moment (write down the actual thoughts). Additionally, note the emotions you felt. To be precise; "mad" is OK but insufficient. Is it a bodily sense, a constriction in the chest, a palpable heartbeat, or a generalized "tense" feeling
Write down your normal "reaction" to that trigger and those associated thoughts and emotions in the Response column. For instance, did you scream the previous time that trigger prompted a response from you, Your voice shook, right? Did you

start acting violently, and if so, how? Did you roll your eyes, leave, and then lash out at someone else later?

Write down your response's immediate beneficial effects in the Positive Consequences column. Typically, this entails the venting of anger as well as momentary gratification or stress reduction. Additionally, try to think of a few long-term advantages (there may not be any of these).

List both the immediate and long-term negative effects in the negative consequences column.

Trigger	Feeling	Response	Negative consequences

Table for recording angry situations

The following are typical short-term negative effects: feeling ashamed after yelling, regretting your dramatic reaction, failing to reach your objective, having people label you as "mad," feeling out of control, experiencing unpleasant bodily sensations, etc. The following are possible long-term negative effects of an angry reaction: relationship harm from recurrent furious outbursts, deterioration of others' trust, and cardiovascular and circulatory system issues brought on by the continuous production of excessive stress hormones.

You'll need to learn new coping mechanisms for handling these triggers, resisting furious thoughts, and calming down without alcohol. Taking a "time out" is one strategy for calming down.

Breathing from your chest won't help you relax; instead, take deep breaths from your diaphragm. Think of your "gut" as the source of your breath. Repeat calming verbs like "relax" or "take it easy" slowly. While taking a deep breath, say it aloud to yourself.

Use pictures to conjure up a tranquil moment from memory or your imagination.

Slow, easy yoga-style movements might help you feel considerably calmer by relaxing your muscles.

Use these methods consistently. When you're in a stressful situation, get used to using them instinctively.

- Managing cravings and thoughts

Your ideas influence what you do. Many times, people are unaware of the power of their ideas. Sometimes, individuals assume they are doing without thinking since these ideas come to them so swiftly. You could observe how your ideas influence your behavior if you could see an immediate replay in slow motion. Drinking may result from three different sorts of ideas, Alcohol-related thoughts or pictures may trigger desires. Examples include visions of bars, ideas about your preferred beverage, and alcoholic odors and noises. These ideas immediately cause cravings. Urges may be sparked by thoughts of alcohol's pleasurable effects. It won't harm me, it'll soothe my anxieties, my friends will think I'm weird if I don't take a drink, it'll help me sleep, or I can only have one, are a few examples. These ideas often focus on the short-term advantages of drinking rather than the potential long-term consequences. Drinking might result from negative thoughts. Additionally, unpleasant feelings and ideas might motivate drinking. These ideas might include feelings of helplessness or low self-worth. Indirect causes include negative thoughts. They create a series of circumstances that may result in drinking.

How to deal with them

1 Consider your reasons for drinking and note any alcohol triggers.

Your worries may be more about why you drink than how much. Many individuals turn to alcohol to dull their emotions or cope with difficult circumstances better. It's typical to drink to ease anxiety before a challenging talk or a first date.

But if you find it difficult to deal with problems without alcohol, you may want to think about whether drinking keeps you from developing more effective coping mechanisms for your emotions.

among the alcohol triggers are

stress in relationships, social gatherings,

working problems and insomnia

You may make plans to help control the impulse to drink by being more aware of your alcohol triggers and motivations.

Inform others about it.

Sharing your decision to quit drinking with others may inspire you to continue with your resolution.
When you quit drinking, your family and friends may encourage you and support you.

Sharing your experiences with alcohol might inspire others to examine their drinking patterns.

Perhaps your spouse, sibling, or roommate is contemplating a shift as well. Together, you can support one another while increasing your drive and accountability by quitting drinking.

fostering community
Developing new connections with those who refrain from drinking might be quite advantageous.

Turner stresses that "the more support you have, the better."

Here are a few concepts:
-Why not ask a different coworker to check out the brand-new bakery down the street instead of putting your resolve to the test by going to the normal happy hour with your colleagues?
-Think about developing relationships with individuals who don't see alcohol use as a high priority in their life.
-Miss the ambiance of the bar? You may be able to go to a sober bar and mingle without drinking depending on where you reside.
-To locate others interested in activities without alcohol, go via applications like Meetup.

-Knowing what to say
People may query you as to why you decline a drink. You're not required to provide specifics, however, it might be useful to be prepared with the following response: "I'm reducing my spending for my health."
I dislike how drinking makes me feel.

Having stated that, all you need to say is "No, thanks." You might feel more at ease and certain when you find yourself in an alcohol-related scenario by practicing your rejection beforehand.
Since the majority of people are unlikely to notice or remember what you do, try not to worry about how others may see you.
Keep your answer straightforward if you want to give loved ones a more thorough explanation but are uncertain of what to say: "I've been drinking a lot lately without really knowing why, and I want to take some time to reconsider that behavior."
"I see that I drink when I don't want to confront my feelings, and I want to get better at processing my emotions without drinking."
I'm sick of drinking simply because everyone else does since I don't like it.
-Change up your routine to stay occupied.
One of the easiest methods to stop a pattern of drinking at a certain time of day is to divert your attention to something else. The most beneficial activities are those that regularly get you outside and moving.

Consider the following:
-Consider taking a walk or meeting your pals for a hangout at the park or another alcohol-free area if you often meet up with friends for drinks after work.
-Why not try a new spot that doesn't offer alcohol instead of heading to your typical restaurant for dinner and drinks? You'll have the opportunity to do something unusual without being tempted to drink.
-To pass the time and save money, make it a practice to cook at home.
Having a few different coping mechanisms available might assist when your urge to drink is more influenced by your mood than any certain time of day:
-Try affirmations, deep breathing exercises, or meditation as alternatives to drinking to reduce anxiety.
-Reach out to a loved one or watch a favorite movie to make yourself feel better when you're feeling lonely.
-Find a new beverage to like.
Making the correct substitution beverage choice might support you in being steadfast in your decision to quit drinking. -Even while plain water has many health advantages, it's not the most exciting option.

You may find something pleasurable to do without missing your favorite beverage if you put a little ingenuity into it.

Try:
-Adding cinnamon or other spices to tea, apple cider, or hot chocolate; infusing plain or sparkling water with chopped fruits or herbs; or combining juice or lemonade with sparkling water

-Eliminate alcohol from your home.
When you're attempting to stop, having alcohol around your home may entice you. Knowing you'll need to go out and make a purchase might dissuade you from taking a drink long enough to locate a suitable diversion.

-Have non-alcoholic drinks available for both you and other people. Being a good host doesn't need you to have to provide the booze. Allow visitors to bring their alcohol, and allow them to take it with them when they go.

-If you share a home with roommates, think about suggesting that they keep their alcohol hidden rather than in common areas.

Chapter 5: Persistent drinking

The National Institute on Alcohol Abuse and Alcoholism estimates that 90% of alcoholics will relapse within four years. Although relapse is quite frequent, it may still be distressing for the individual and seem like a significant setback on the journey to recovery. Relapse, however, need not lead to a full-blown addiction again.

People in recovery from alcoholism relapse for a variety of reasons. Stress or exposure to events that they identify with the euphoric sensation previously caused by alcohol might trigger some individuals. Others turn to alcohol again to deal with underlying anxiety, despair, or persistent pain.

If you discover that you have relapsed, it is essential to first acknowledge that it occurred before figuring out how to go on. Create a plan to prevent relapsing in the future and let go of the guilt and humiliation related to the mistake.

Relapse prevention is a key component of long-term relapse management strategies. The following tactics are successful in lowering relapse chances for those who are dependent on alcohol or another substance.

-Avoiding certain people, locations, and objects. avoiding the people, locations, and circumstances that formerly prompted the individual to use alcohol or other drugs.

-Using both clinical and non-clinical assistance as necessary.

-A robust support system, whether it be formalized by a service provider or unofficially by a group of encouraging friends and family, will aid in preventing undesirable behaviors and circumstances.

engaging in worthwhile tasks.

-Encourage the individual to develop a good sense of self-image and pride by engaging in activities they like and that benefit the neighborhood, such as joining a local athletic team, choir, or special interest club.

-Balanced living and self-care: Substance use may be triggered by failing to take care of one's physical and mental health.

Reasons for relapse which you would love to prevent

Several situations might encourage relapse.

-Conditions or locations where the individual would have previously used alcohol or another drug, for example, are situations that entice the person to resume drug use.
-Situations that cause people to take drugs as a coping mechanism, such as unstable housing, failure in their careers or personal lives, peer pressure, or societal shame. existing emotional or mental health problems.
-Underlying physical health conditions. Some persons with poor physical health may turn to over-the-counter pharmaceuticals, especially if they have chronic pain. Guilt brought on a relapse: A person who is attempting to stop using drugs or alcohol could feel conflicted or guilty if they fail. If this issue is not handled correctly, it may result in feelings of shame and self-blame, which increases the likelihood that the individual will continue using drugs or alcohol as a coping technique.
You can get back on track and overcome your relapse by doing the below actions.

- Immediately stop drinking.
People who have a history of alcohol use disorder (AUD) often remain drinking after relapsing. They believe there is no purpose in quitting because they have messed up. However, if you keep drinking, it will become more difficult to quit, which will reinforce your addiction.

One of the most crucial things you can do after a relapse, according to addiction specialist Lin Sternlicht, LMHC, MA, EdM, is to quit as soon as you can. "It will be simpler to go on the better you can manage your relapse in terms of amount and length."

-Look for help
Nobody can overcome addiction on their own. To get the support you need to avoid future relapses, enlist the assistance of trustworthy family members and friends.

-Twelve-step organizations like Alcoholics Anonymous may be highly beneficial because they provide a secure setting for sharing and learning from others' experiences with recovery. You may find treatment choices, including alcohol rehab and AUD meds, with the assistance of a qualified addiction counselor.

-Determine your triggers.
Triggers are stimuli that make you want to drink or use drugs again, sometimes resulting in relapse. They may range from being around individuals who misuse alcohol to going to areas that remind you of drinking, going through stressful circumstances, or even eating specific things.

-Knowing your triggers can enable you to avoid or reduce circumstances that could lead to relapse. You may employ coping mechanisms like logic to resist temptation when a trigger is present. You may identify your triggers and create coping mechanisms for them with the assistance of a qualified therapist who specializes in drug use disorders.

According to psychotherapist Dmitri Oster, LCSW, CASAC II, "the more attentive to one's relapse triggers a client is, the more they may understand those triggers and become empowered to not let them undermine their recovery efforts in the present and future."

4. Create a strategy to avoid relapsing once again.
Try to assess your relapse and formulate a strategy to prevent a similar situation in the future with the aid of a therapist, a qualified addiction counselor, or a sponsor. This should include potential triggers, coping mechanisms, and particular members of your support system that you may turn to for assistance.

-Risk of overdose during relapse
Regular drug users build up a tolerance to the substance, which means they need to take more of it to have the same effect. A person's tolerance to the medicine may decrease if they don't take it for a period. As a result, when individuals resume taking their customary dosage after a break, the body may not be able to handle it and an overdose may result.

People who take drugs again after a break run a special risk of overdose owing to altered tolerance. For instance, upon a release from custody and during detox and/or rehabilitation. For instance, someone on naltrexone may put themselves in danger if they use it shortly after finishing their oral medicine, if they miss a dosage, or after the benefits of their implanted naltrexone have worn off.

Immediately seek medical help if an overdose is suspected.

Additional measures for vulnerable people

A person may need to use extra techniques to aid recovery and ward off relapse if they are dealing with chronic emotional, physical, and/or mental health problems.

-Finding the ideal combination of drugs, such as antidepressants or anxiety relievers - the individual should see their general practitioner or psychiatrist to locate a drug that works for them.

Alternative strategies, such as yoga, mindfulness-based treatments, or meditation, promote a more comprehensive approach to wellbeing

-Psychological assistance, such as psychotherapy, CBT, or drug or alcohol treatment

Creating dietary, exercise, and sleep regimens for oneself.

another successful relapse prevention strategy

Slips may be quite difficult. You could encounter difficulties even while employing your greatest abilities. It will be easier for you in the long term if you don't, but despite your best efforts, it's conceivable that you'll finally have a drink. When they relapse, some individuals give up on their attempts to abstain from alcohol. If drinking does take place, it's crucial to understand that a single drink doesn't always definitely result in a full-blown relapse. When one slips, one might consider the following three options: -

-The error shouldn't be made again. If the individual stops drinking after this, it is seen as a lapse.

-The slip provides a chance to learn about a perilous situation. The individual should consider other strategies for handling the circumstance in the future. If the individual does not continue drinking but instead learns a lesson for the future, this is referred to as a "prolapse."

-The accident is a catastrophe that demonstrates the person's helplessness. People who see the slide in this manner believe they have failed. I'll never be successful. I'm simply going to give up. Relapsing means giving up and picking up drinking again. The worst option is the third way of thinking. Slips are comparable to falling off a bike. Even though it can hurt, you should get back up on your bike and continue riding. Even though you may feel terrible about your slip-up, you may still resume your sobriety. The mistake might even provide a chance to gain knowledge about a challenging circumstance.

A slip may be avoided by observing warning signals and considering them. Even those who make a concerted effort to abstain from alcohol and other drugs sometimes run into difficult circumstances. We think you should be ready for a slip even if you should work hard and anticipate not having another drink. You have options if you decide to drink. As was previously said, there are three diverse perspectives on the beverage. You may see it as an error (a slip), an error from which you can learn (a prolapse), or as a catastrophic failure (a relapse). To never relapse is the objective. It's not necessary to relapse after having a drink. If you ever consume alcohol, attempt to make it seem like prolapse or slip. If you drink, keep these things in mind:

1. Remain calm. One drink does not always signal the start of a long binge or a return to reckless drinking.

2. Pause, gaze, and pay attention. Stop the current course of action, glance around, and pay attention to what is going on. The lapse needs to be seen as a red flag indicating the client or couple may be in jeopardy. It is necessary to stop off the road to address the lapse like a flat tire.

3. Recognize the impact of abstinence violations. After consuming alcohol, you can think, "I blew it," "All our efforts were in vain," "As long as I've blown it, I might as well keep drinking," or "My willpower has failed, I have no control," or "I'm hooked, and once I drink, my body will take over." Feelings of rage or guilt may accompany these ideas. It is essential to instantly refute these ideas.

4.Reaffirm your dedication. It is simple to get disheartened and desire to quit after a slip-up. Consider the factors that led you to decide to modify your drinking in the first place. Examine your decisional matrix and consider all the long-term advantages of quitting drinking as well as all the issues that would arise if you continued to do so. 5. Choose a course of action :This should at the very least involve: Leaving the drinking environment. Delaying a second drink for at least two hours. Preventing further drinking throughout those two hours by engaging in some activity. The activity may be enjoyable, include reading treatment materials, involve discussing the lapse with a person who could be helpful, involve phoning your therapist, or involve any combination of these.

6. Examine the circumstances that led up to the lapse. You are not to blame for what occurred. You will feel more guilty and guilty about yourself if you concentrate on your own mistakes. What circumstances lead up to the mistake, you could ask? What were the primary causes? Were there any early symptoms of trouble? Did you attempt to resolve them positively? Why not, then? Were you demotivated due to exhaustion, peer pressure, or depression? After you have examined the slide, consider the adjustments you should do to prevent other slips.

7. Seek assistance. Asking someone to support you, encourage you, provide you with advise, divert you, or engage in a different activity with you will make things simpler for you. The same thing would apply if you had a flat tire and your spare tire was also flat: you would need assistance. Write out some strategies for dealing with slips or relapses if they happen using the worksheet that is given.

Chapter 5: Look how far you have come

This will show you the "big picture" of the treatment plan, show you how far along you are, and show you how many new abilities you now possess. In the course of therapy, you have already learned a lot. You have been honing a variety of techniques to assist you to refrain from drinking. You have a greater understanding of alcohol in terms of typical drinks, blood alcohol content, and problematic drinking levels. You have been self-recording, becoming aware of your triggers, and understanding the sequence of events that leads to drinking when one of your triggers is present. You now know what environmental signals may cause you to feel or think in a manner that leads to drinking. Knowing which dangerous scenarios would test you the most has allowed you to prepare since knowledge is power. And now that you know these scenarios are coming up in advance, you can make the necessary plans. Before it gets out of hand, you'll be able to spot the problem coming. You've looked at your social network and identified possible drinking triggers as well as nondrinkers who may act as protective barriers for you. To be ready with a precise response for each trigger, you've learned to create strategies for dealing with them. You have weighed the benefits and drawbacks of abstinence and drinking to be more convinced that the benefits of abstinence exceed those of drinking. You are also more aware of the drawbacks of alcohol use. You now have some new strategies for overcoming cravings and temptations. You now know the several categories of negative emotions and their signs. You're moving forward! Stay tuned because you'll be learning how to:

-Calm yourself when you're worried or depressed
- Speak up
-Replace drinking's positive consequences with sobriety's negative ones
-Challenge problematic alcohol-related thoughts
-Deal effectively with situations where alcohol is present
-Make less risky decisions
-Solve problems effectively
-Better manage your anger.
Recognize the precursors to relapses, avoid them, and cope with any slips.

www.ingramcontent.com/pod-product-compliance
Lightning Source LLC
LaVergne TN
LVHW080559160826
845677LV00010B/1909

* 9 7 9 8 3 6 8 1 8 1 8 9 9 *